"I'm Not Dead Yet"

Living Every Moment

by Mary Gatschene

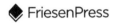

Suite 300 - 990 Fort St
Victoria, BC, V8V 3K2
Canada

www.friesenpress.com

Copyright © 2017 by Mary Gatschene
First Edition — 2017

Some names and identifying details have been changed to protect the privacy of individuals.

ISBN
978-1-5255-0024-4 (Hardcover)
978-1-5255-0025-1 (Paperback)
978-1-5255-0026-8 (eBook)

1. MEDICAL, NURSING

Distributed to the trade by The Ingram Book Company

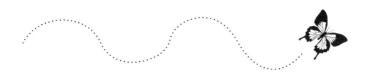

ACKNOWLEDGEMENTS

I would like to express my thanks to all the people who have given me the opportunity to care for them and share their stories. To Marybeth, who gave life to the caregiver in this book. To all the caregivers, both professional and non-professional, who work so diligently to provide excellent end-of-life care to those in need. To an exceptional physician, Dr. Ward, who inspired me to even consider writing this book. To my life-long friend, Suzanne, who graciously allowed me to share her picture on the cover. To my cherished editor and sister, Donna, who encouraged and supported me through this journey. When my menopausal brain shut down and the words were lost, she was there to find them and give this project finesse—what a team! To my greatest supporter, my soulmate and husband, Gary, who listened patiently to every story I wrote, over and over again, with praise and encouragement. I love you for sharing this new endeavour with me.

TABLE OF CONTENTS

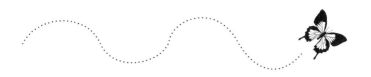

INTRODUCTION

This book was written for everyone who has experienced the loss of a loved one, in the hopes that they have also experienced the joy and peace which can be found in living every moment at the end of life.

I am a Registered Nurse who specializes in palliative care. I have worked in different palliative care settings including some hospices in Canada. The length of stay of residents I have cared for in hospice has been from one hour to four months.

When hearing the word "hospice," many people think of an environment that is dark and depressing. The reality is that a hospice can be a place of laughter, great memories, comfort and love. There are many happy moments in hospice that are important to those who are on their final journey in life. Our residents come to hospice not to "die" but to "live until they die." There is meaning to everything we do, from living to dying. If we can embrace the idea that we are not able to live forever, that dying is something we share with the human race, then perhaps we can come to terms with our fate and live each moment until that day.

I was inspired by a comment that came from one of my residents on her admission to the hospice. Her family arrived with her and they were distressed and in tears. She looked at me and said, with a little smile and a wink, "I'm not dead yet"; thus the title of this book. Just because our residents are dying doesn't mean they can't share some meaningful conversations or live every moment while they are able to. We, as caregivers, have the opportunity to assist them in accomplishing their goals and completing their legacy—to learn who they are and why they are so loved.

People ask me, "How can you work in such a sad and depressing environment?" Well, firstly, I don't believe it's depressing at all, and once you read the stories I think you will see that, too. I believe that those of us who work in hospice have been given a special gift—a gift of compassion for those at the end of their life—and we need to cherish this gift and pass it forward to those in need. Do I find this specialized field of nursing worth it when I go home emotionally and physically drained? Yes, because I have the opportunity to meet some of the most amazing people, and I am honoured to be able to care for them, give them comfort and be a part of their lives, even for a short time. We can learn so much from those who think they have nothing left to give.

I'm Not Dead Yet—Living Every Moment describes some of the precious, happy moments that I have experienced with my residents, patients and their families

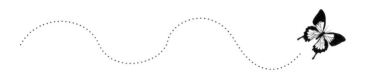

WHERE TO START

It is very important to determine what a resident's level of understanding is about their illness before developing a plan of care. Some residents, when admitted to hospice, think they are there to get better treatment because their doctor told them the current treatment is not working or they no longer require it (in other words, the chemotherapy is not working because the tumor has spread to other areas). Some think they are there to get stronger by receiving physiotherapy (thinking it's a rehabilitation centre) so they can return to their home. It is important that residents and their families understand that the goal of hospice is not to improve the resident's health, but to provide pain and symptom management during their natural progressive decline.

One definition of palliative care is "an approach that improves the quality of life of a person and their family facing the issues associated with life-threatening illness." We, as caregivers, reach out to cloak them, to cover them with loving care and protect them.

Getting to know our residents not by the diseases they have but by who they are as a person helps to affirm their sense of importance and give them the feeling of being a unique individual. It maintains their sense of dignity. The end of life is a time for people to reflect on how they want to be remembered by those who will cherish their legacy.

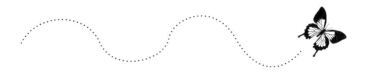

MARYBETH

Marybeth represents all the caregivers in this book. To make the stories flow together, I decided to give the caregiver one name so everyone who has provided care for a loved one could identify with her.

The name I chose was Marybeth. She was actually one of my patients, and she taught me so much about hope and coping. Marybeth was deaf, so that presented a challenge for me because I did not know sign language and I was concerned about how to communicate with her. I knew I had to be creative to properly assess her pain and symptoms, so we made up our own sign language and wrote pages and pages of notes. It took time, but we mastered it very well.

Marybeth always had a smile on her face when I visited her, even when she was not feeling well. She often wore a pink hat, as she had lost her hair after receiving chemotherapy. The hat brought out the glow in her face. At each visit, we would review the list of symptoms, and she would rate them on a scale of zero to ten. Often, with a grin, she would say her pain was a ten out of ten just to see if I was paying attention. Some days I think we both had cramps in our hands from all our writing, as we both had so much to say with the non-medical dialogue as we caught up on what was happening in our lives.

Marybeth's visits were always around the same time of day. Because she could not hear the doorbell, we would get a key from the lockbox at her house and let ourselves in. I remember one visit when I walked in and found her sleeping in the La-Z-Boy chair. I knew she couldn't hear me, and I didn't want to alarm her by touching her arm to awaken her, so I stood there for a moment trying to decide what to do. All of a sudden she jumped and scared the living daylights out of me. With a twinkle in her eyes and a huge grin on her face, she wrote down that she had seen me coming but kept her eyes closed so she could give me a scare. Did she ever!

Marybeth had a great sense of humour, and her smile would brighten up even the worst day. Every visit ended with a hug and a wave goodbye. We shared good times when she was feeling well and bad times when she was nauseated or fatigued from her chemotherapy and just wanted to stay in bed. Even when she decided to stop the chemotherapy because the cancer was progressing and she had to come to terms with the reality of dying, she stayed focused on living and enjoying each day. After every visit, I would leave her house so inspired. I remember the day she died. As she was taking her last breaths, I held her hand and whispered in her ear, "Go with the angels, Marybeth. They are waiting for you." She actually got a little smile on her face. Talking to her seemed so natural, and I forgot that she probably could not hear what I said. Perhaps in that moment she did hear me and that is why she smiled. I think she heard the angels calling her!

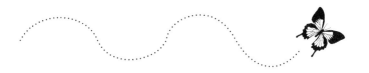

MY PERSONAL STORY

My personal story, which empowered me to impress upon people the importance of living every moment, occurred when I was thirty years old. I missed the chance to say goodbye to one of my best friends before she died.

Lisa had cystic fibrosis, and during the last few years of her life she was often admitted to hospital due to lung infections. Many of our visits occurred in the hospital cafeteria as we walked along pushing her intravenous pole, or in her hospital room where we would sit and drink tea and laugh about the good old days when we were in nursing together.

I had promised her, and myself, that I would be with her when she got worse and was dying, as we knew would happen. I told my husband that whatever was going on in our lives at the time did not matter because I needed to be with Lisa when that time came.

I remember coming home one morning from night shift and my husband telling me to call Lisa's husband. When I called, he told me that Lisa had died in his arms overnight. I was devastated! I felt angry that they had not called to tell me how sick she was. Her husband said Lisa did not want him to call me because she didn't want me to see her "that way." I felt angry that I was not given the chance to tell her how much I loved her and that I would never forget her. I lost the chance to say goodbye.

I thought I would be able to cope because I was a nurse, after all, and I knew what the stages of grief were. I was wrong. I thought I could pass by some of the stages, like anger, and be fine. Wrong again. My four-year-old daughter would find me crying and say, "Don't worry, Mommy, some day you will be able to sit and have a cup of tea with Lisa in heaven."

I was distressed for many months, and then one night I had a dream. Lisa and I were standing in the forest, talking about everyday things, when I suddenly noticed that her cheeks were rosy and her blonde hair was glowing. (In life she was quite pale.) I realized at that moment that she was dead and started to cry, saying to her, "Lisa, you are dead!" She answered, "Yes, and I feel great." I asked her why her husband was coping better than I was, and she replied that he had witnessed her suffering and was able to find closure after being with her through the dying process. She had the most beautiful smile as she spoke to me. That's when I woke up. I truly believe that Lisa had come to me in my dreams to say goodbye.

After that night I felt peaceful and was able to heal and continue with my life, which I value as more precious than ever before. I regret not telling Lisa often enough how important she was to me and how she had enriched my life. I now tell those I love just how much I love them and always say goodbye with a hug. We don't always have the time or opportunity to say goodbye to those we love, so when we do we should embrace those moments and make them a reality.

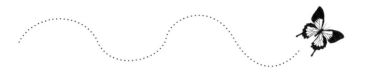

A PRIVATE BEACH

Janine was a close friend of mine. We met at a sports event with our children and became inseparable. She was battling cancer and was determined to fight to the end. At the time, I was working at a hospital and did not have much experience with palliative care. Janine's dream was to take a trip to Cuba with her husband and spend time on the beach. She followed all her doctor's instructions so she could be as healthy as possible and be allowed to travel. Her family was very supportive and made the arrangements, planning for everything that could come up while she was there. She was given approval by her medical team for this last trip before she became too sick.

One week before she was to leave, Janine developed a complication due to her cancer and became quite ill. Her trip to Cuba had to be canceled. She knew there would not be another chance to go.

She had lost the window of opportunity to fulfill her dream.

I wanted to do something special for Janine to show that I cared about her loss. I knew it was not the destination Janine longed for, but to feel the warm sand on her skin. The beach represented relaxation—a place to forget her troubles and feel the warmth of the sun with her husband close by.

I filled a small box with beach sand from my own family's cottage. I glued pictures to foam backing— pictures of flip flops, an umbrella, a towel, a book, a strawberry daiquiri, a lawn chair, sunscreen and sunglasses. I included a miniature toy rake, beach ball, pail and shovel from a toy store and made a sign saying "Janine's beach. Admittance permission required."

I gave the box to Janine, stating that now she had her own private beach to visit whenever she wanted. She could play in the sand and use the rake to find all the things she would need at the beach, and she could invite whoever she wanted to accompany her. I even included a free pass for her husband. Janine cried and hugged me. She said she was probably the only person who had her own private beach and would enjoy it every day, which she did until her death several weeks later.

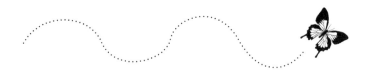

AN INNOCENT SLIP
OF THE TONGUE

Everyone has phrases they repeat that can have several meanings; for example, "break a leg," which can mean "good luck." Today's teenagers may label something "sick," which actually means "that's really cool." We widely use these double-meaning phrases without even thinking about them. If it is a quiet shift at work, someone may remark, "Boy, it's really dead tonight!" Or a staff member coming on night shift who did not sleep well may lament, "I am so dead tired tonight." When repositioning someone in bed you may say, "I'm going to help you go to the other side" when you actually mean "I'm going to help you turn on your other side."

These are not good things to say if you work at a hospice.

One evening, Marybeth was assisting her co-worker to get John settled for bed. He was very drowsy this particular evening and was asleep before they finished tidying up his room. Marybeth emptied urine from his catheter into a plastic measuring container and placed the container on the floor, then leaned forward to say "Goodnight, John, have a good sleep."

Her co-worker, seeing the container of urine on the floor near Marybeth's foot, warned, "Don't kick the bucket." Marybeth looked up in horror when she heard this, then realized with relief that her co-worker was speaking to her, not John, who was sound asleep. In that particular case, "Don't kick the bucket" meant, literally, just that.

Sometimes these one-liners are expressed by those in our care, and it gives us an opportunity to discuss what is most concerning to them about dying. One of my patients told me he was going to be admitted to hospice because his "time was up," another said he had "one foot in the grave," and a third said there was "nothing left for me now but a pine box." Each of these cases gave me the perfect opportunity to question my patients about how they felt about this, opening up the discussion to what their fears were, how they understood the dying process and what their goals were for pain and symptom management. These conversations are critical, but often difficult to initiate, as the dying person usually doesn't want to burden their family with such conversations.

Until we can understand what the palliative patient's priorities are going forward, that is, their goals of care, it is difficult to assist them in fulfilling their legacy. We need to respect their end-of-life decisions and be their advocate in assisting family members to do the same, thus allowing them to maintain their dignity. Living every moment is not just about the special happy moments we can provide, but also about redirecting our patients' energy towards emotional and psychological acceptance of their journey so they are able to fully enjoy those special moments. I like to explain to those in my care that it is important to discuss the difficult topics and then file them away on a shelf and start to live the rest of their lives. Not everyone will come to accept where their journey is leading them, but we will continue to reach out to them with compassion and acceptance to provide them with an environment of serenity.

So please, excuse your caregivers if we inadvertently make a comment that seems inappropriate in a hospice setting. We, too, are only human and we can sometimes put our foot in our mouth. Besides,

I wouldn't be caught dead saying something that would be misinterpreted......Oops!

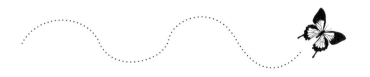

JUST ONE MORE SMOKE

As many as 85% of our residents develop delirium at the end of life. They may hallucinate, and their reality is often distorted. To them, an experience is real, and if you tell them it is not real, they may become more agitated. Comforting them is of utmost importance. They require a calm, quiet environment and a gentle and caring approach.

Randy was a lovely gentleman who came to the hospice with lung cancer. He had smoked cigarettes most of his adult life and had "quit" many times but always returned to what he referred to as "that nasty habit."

His family would take him outside in his wheelchair to the designated smoking area, but, as he became weaker and had more breathing difficulties, he could no longer handle this "trip to the smokehouse."

As his health deteriorated, Randy became delirious. Even though he wore a nicotine patch, he missed having a cigarette between his fingers. He told Marybeth that someone had stolen his cigarettes and he became more and more agitated as he searched unsuccessfully through his bed. Marybeth wanted to ease his distress but knew she could not allow him to smoke in his room. She cut a drinking straw in half, stuffed a cotton ball in the end of it, then gave it to Randy, explaining that it was a new kind of cigarette. He looked at it and then thanked her. Just when she thought he was settling, he asked , "Have you got a light?" Marybeth told Randy she would be right back, then quickly took the "cigarette" to the nursing station where she used a red marker to color the end of the cotton ball. Returning to his room, she handed him the straw saying, "Here, I lit it for you." He put it to his mouth and proceeded to "smoke" the cigarette. He was given a plastic bowl for an ashtray and he gently tapped the straw on the edge, knocking off the imaginary ashes.

Whenever Randy requested a "smoke", the staff would give him his special cigarette, already "lit." With his medication for delirium and his cigarette between his fingers, Randy spent many a day safely in his bed, smoking, and not once was there found to be a burn hole in the sheets.

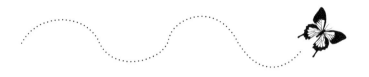

A PRECIOUS KISS

Hospice can be a wonderful alternative for family members, as hospice staff take over the care of their loved one, allowing them to now be the spouse, mother, father, son or daughter without the worry of having to be the caregiver as well. Hospice allows family members to get a good night's rest at home and get re-energized for the difficult time ahead. It allows them to spend quality time with their loved one and create those precious moments that are so important.

When a lovely lady, Merla, was diagnosed with cancer, her family wanted to care for her and allow her to die at home. Unfortunately, it became too difficult, so Merla was admitted to a residential hospice, where she spent her last week.

When residents are admitted to hospice, our care and compassion must also be for the families they bring with them. Special attention is often required for children involved in this life-changing event called "death."

Merla was very close to her eight-year-old grand-daughter, Summer. Summer understood that her Nana was going to die. Her family, realizing the importance of including her in Nana's last journey, allowed Summer to stay home from school one day a week to help care for her.

Marybeth wanted to give Summer a lasting memory of her Nana- something precious to comfort her and remind her of her Nana's love. She and Summer rolled and cut out a clay heart, then cut a smaller heart from inside it. They carried the small heart to Nana's room where they helped Nana, (as she was unconscious) to kiss her index finger and then place that kiss in the middle of the small heart. Summer then decorated the larger heart , making an "N" for Nana with purple beads, her Nana's favorite color.

Summer was very excited to know that she was the only one with a kiss from her Nana that she would have forever. Marybeth pierced a hole in the small heart so Summer could wear it as a necklace. At night Summer could take it off and place it inside the larger heart for safe-keeping.. She wore her precious necklace at the celebration of Merla's life and would occasionally hold the heart in her hand. Summer was told that whenever she missed her Nana she could touch the heart and feel Nana's kiss and know that she was close by watching over her.

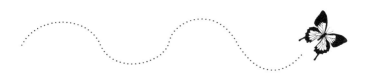

HIGH TEA FOR YOU AND ME

Elizabeth, a very classy British lady, was admitted to hospice. Before her illness, she and her girlfriends would meet for "high tea" every month. They all lived out of town, so would gather halfway at a cozy little tea house. Elizabeth told Marybeth that their last tea party had been about three months ago, and that she wished she could visit again with her friends. She had spoken to each of them by phone in the past few months, but missed the times when they were all together, sharing their lives with each other and solving the problems of the world.

One of Elizabeth's friends called the hospice regularly for updates, so, during one of these conversations, Marybeth suggested that they plan a surprise "high tea" social for the group of friends. The friend eagerly agreed, and invitations were sent to all the ladies.

On the day of the tea, Marybeth gave Elizabeth her own invitation. Assuming the tea was for all the hospice residents, Elizabeth stated, "I don't have any other plans, so I guess I will go."

The hospice staff had decorated a table in the sunroom with china dishes and a white tablecloth. The kitchen staff had prepared small sandwiches and special bite-sized desserts. A local lady volunteered to play the harp during "high tea."

When Elizabeth was escorted into the sunroom in her wheelchair by a porter dressed in a black suit and chauffer's cap, she cried out in delight to see all her friends at the table with smiles on their faces.

The ladies enjoyed an afternoon of tea and friendship. They discussed the joys and sorrows of their lives and made a promise to each other to meet again one day in heaven. They agreed that the first one there had to set up the tea table and wait for the others to arrive. Elizabeth said that, since she would be the first one, she would have everything ready, but told them to hurry along before the tea got too cold. They all smiled and lifted their teacups to toast their dear friend.

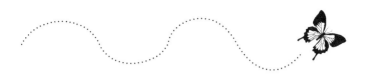

A DANCE WITH MY DAUGHTER

John was a fifty-seven-year-old man who came to hospice after a short battle with cancer. He was very distressed because his daughter was getting married in two months, but his prognosis was less than one month. John had always dreamed of the day he would proudly dance with his daughter at her wedding; now he likely would not even be alive for the special day. Melissa was his only child and had always been "daddy's little girl." As a child, she had followed him everywhere. Every morning, she would peel back his eyelids, saying, "Wake up now, daddy."

When Melissa voiced the same concerns about the wedding to Marybeth, the hospice team discussed how they could possibly fulfill this last wish for John. Marybeth spoke to an instructor who taught ballroom dancing at a local studio and, together with John's wife and daughter, they came up with a plan.

On the chosen day, hospice staff decorated the lounge. Melissa brought a recording of the song she had selected for the dance with her father, and John's wife brought a friend to videotape the special event. John's wife helped him get dressed in the suit he was planning to wear to his daughter's wedding, telling him they were going to attend a hospice event.

John was taken to the lounge in his wheelchair, where he found his daughter waiting in her wedding dress. Melissa sat on her dad's lap as the song "Dance with My Father" began to play. The tuxedoed dance instructor took the handles of the wheelchair and began to gently twirl and glide the couple around the room. As Melissa and John smilingly "danced", there was not a dry eye in the room.

Melissa told her dad that a part of him would be with her on her wedding day, and his spirit would live on in her. She would show this video to her future children and tell them all about her loving father. John glanced at Marybeth, mouthing the words "Thank you" with tears in his eyes.

John died a few weeks later. At her wedding, Melissa played the video after the first dance with her groom, projecting it on a large screen so all her guests could watch. Melissa will forever cherish the memory of those special moments with her dad.

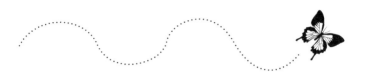

BAKING DAY WITH GRANDMA

Patricia lived for her grandchildren. She planned special events with each of them at various ages. When each grandchild turned six years old , he or she would have a "baking day with Grandma." They would spend hours rolling out and decorating sugar cookies together. Patricia always had a ready supply of colorful sprinkles and candy shapes to add to the cookies before baking them.

Patricia was admitted to hospice with lung cancer after trying unsuccessfully to remain at home. Due to increased weakness and fatigue, she decided she could no longer care for herself. Her youngest grandchild, Stephanie, would be turning six years old in three months, and Patricia felt like she had failed her, because she would be the only grandchild who would not have had a "baking day with Grandma." She felt guilty and wished that she could have "tried harder" to stay at home and "hang in there" a little longer.

Marybeth spoke with Patricia's daughter, Susie, about making this tradition happen for her mother and Stephanie. On the arranged day, Susie brought in the ingredients for the prized sugar cookie recipe, and Marybeth provided the utensils. Stephanie, dressed in a chef's hat and apron, walked into Patricia's room carrying a mixing bowl. She asked Grandma if she was ready to bake cookies with her. Patricia hugged Stephanie as tears rolled down her face.

Together, grandmother and granddaughter mixed up a batch of cookies. They rolled out the dough and cut out angel shapes -- Stephanie's choice as she knew Grandma was going to be an angel some day. They laughed as they decorated the cookies with sprinkles brought from Patricia's cupboard at home. Then, while Patricia rested, Stephanie watched Marybeth bake the cookies.

When the cookies were ready, Stephanie carried them to Patricia's room for a tea party with cookies and milk. While they sat together, dipping their cookies in their glass of milk, they shared the memories that were captured on film of the special "baking day with Grandma."

Patricia told Marybeth that she always wanted to be fair to all her grandchildren because each one had a special place in her heart. She said that if something was important enough, then it was worth the effort of creating that special memory with the help of caring people. Now she could rest assured that she had left each grandchild with a special moment in time.

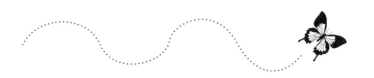

A MOVIE NIGHT—OR TWO

Tiffany loved to watch movies. When she was well, she would go to the movies every two weeks with her children. They would buy the biggest bag of popcorn and share it. With all those little hands in the bag, Tiffany rarely got more than a few handfuls, but she loved every moment. As her children got older they continued the movie night, taking turns deciding which movie to see.

Since becoming so ill with cancer, Tiffany's movie nights came to an end. She sadly reminisced about how those times brought her closer to her children as everyone sat in their seats concentrating on the action on the screen, silent (except for an excited word here or there followed by a whispered, "Shhh") and anticipating what would happen next. Now she was lying in bed, slowly dying of cancer and running out of time to spend with her family.

Tiffany's three children were now between the ages of 10 and 14. They also reminisced about those special movie nights with their mom. Marybeth talked to Tiffany about planning a movie night at the hospice with her children, but Tiffany sadly admitted that she didn't think she had the energy to stay awake for the entire movie, especially in the evening. Marybeth suggested, "Why not watch the movie over two nights? You could have a contest with the children to see who can come closest to guessing what will happen at the end, and the winner will get a prize!" Tiffany smiled and said, "Let's do it. The kids will love it!"

Marybeth was able to borrow a large portable screen, and the hospice team provided popcorn, drinks and candy. The children were told that they would watch the first hour of the movie on Saturday afternoon, then they had to guess how the movie would end. After they finished watching on Sunday afternoon, their mom would decide the winner. Tiffany's youngest child chose the movie "Dunston Checks In."

The three children sat in and around Tiffany's bed, cuddled up in their own private theatre. Tiffany smiled as she looked down and saw many hands in the popcorn bowl. Marybeth was able to get some free movie passes as prizes for all the children because, of course, each child guessed the correct ending to the movie.

Tiffany later told Marybeth that it was a very special weekend and thanked everyone for their help in making her "movie night" become more than a last wish. She cherished the photos taken by hospice staff of her children enjoying this time with her.

Many families have special traditions that bring their family closer together and which are continued with each new generation. It is not always a once-a-year tradition like having Christmas dinner at Grandma's house. These traditions are often something much easier to accomplish with a little imagination and creativity, like a movie night with mom, creating cherished memories for all.

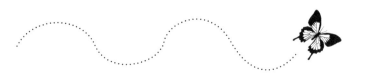

EVERYONE DESERVES
SOME COMFORT

On a medical mission to Peru, South America, the poverty that I witnessed was heartbreaking. I felt that if I was able to help make the life of just one person more comfortable, then I had accomplished a goal. I believe everyone can make a difference by helping one person at a time. Everyone deserves compassion and comfort at the end of life, regardless of where they live.

On this mission trip, I met a family whose daughter was dying. She was about twenty-seven years old and weighed only about 100 pounds. She lay on a bed of wooden boards covered with black garbage bags. Her family asked our team if there was anything we could do to help their daughter. Unfortunately, there was nothing we could do medically to save her, although we were able to provide a limited supply of pain medication. Privately, our team discussed what we could do to help make a difference in the time she had left to live. Quickly, a plan came together.

We hired a local "tuk tuk" (a type of taxi-- a three-wheeled canopied motorcycle with a double – seated cart attached) to take us to a local store where we were able to purchase a mattress. We then drove to the girl's house, with the mattress firmly tied to the top of the taxi. We gently lifted her up, placed the mattress on the wooden boards and made up the bed with sheets we had brought to use at our clinic. When the girl lay back down on the bed, her family stood around crying tears of joy. We were able to at least make her last days more comfortable. We later learned that she had lived for several months, and her family cared for her with the same compassion and love that we would show our own family members.

I feel so fortunate to live in a country where palliative care/ hospice care is an important part of our culture and is accessible to those suffering life-limiting illnesses. We are blessed to have educated and experienced caregivers to provide the services required to care for our loved ones.

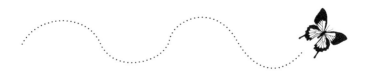

A GIFT FOR MY GIRLS

Susan was one of the most precious and loving women I have ever met. She always had a smile for everyone and was surrounded by people who loved her. Her progressive disease left her with fine motor control difficulties and as she deteriorated she required assistance with eating and personal care.

Susan had two beautiful daughters, Lauren and Morgan, whom she adored. Her husband and the girls would visit her after school most days and they would enjoy family time together before the girls had to go home to their dreaded homework.

At this time, a well-known artist was visiting the hospice. He also happened to be a friend of Susan's mother. Susan had often spoken about her wish to create a hand-made gift to leave for her daughters, so Marybeth mentioned this desire to the artist. He generously offered to donate his time and art supplies to help Susan paint a picture for each girl.

Marybeth and her coworkers set up a table by Susan's bed so she could work comfortably. Together she and the artist created a painting of two ships passing in the night, the artist guiding her hand when Susan found it too difficult to control the paintbrush. Marybeth and the other hospice staff would often stop by the room to watch as Susan's work of art covered the canvas.

Although Susan was growing more exhausted, she was determined to complete a second painting before she ran out of time. Again the artist assisted her and they painted a snowy winter scene. He then took away both canvases to be framed at his own expense.

When the paintings were ready, they were displayed in Susan's room. Everyone knew how much effort it had taken for Susan to paint the two canvases, and the pride in her face was evident as she looked at her work. Her daughters were amazed at their mother's strength and persistence in meeting her goal of giving them a gift from her heart.

Susan spent her life giving to others in everything from her job to her family to her friends. She loved life and lived for every moment, even at the end of life.

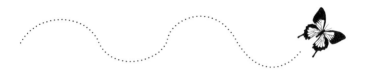

MEMORIES OF AUTUMN

Ellen loved autumn. It was her favourite season. Growing up she enjoyed preparing for Thanksgiving dinner and decorating the house with colorful leaves and pumpkins. In the spring of one year, she was diagnosed with an aggressive form of cancer and spent many months either running to chemotherapy treatments or recovering from the side effects of those treatments. After many long months, she was told that the chemotherapy was not working and that nothing more could be done to treat her cancer.

Ellen spent weeks trying to absorb what was happening to her and, because she felt so unwell, her "list of things to do before I die" was the least of her priorities. She was admitted to a hospice after spending time at home trying to decide what needed to be taken care of before she died. It had been a slow process, as she was experiencing fatigue daily and found it difficult to concentrate.

Once at the hospice, she had time to think and was mourning the fact that she had wasted the previous months trying to settle all her affairs and not really living the rest of her life. She had not spent any time thinking of her autumn and Thanksgiving celebration, which would be her last one. She was restricted to bed, and it was not possible to go for her yearly walk in the forest to pick leaves or to the family pumpkin patch to collect various pumpkins to carve. She could only look out the window and dream of the last time she was able to enjoy being in nature surrounded by colorful leaves.

One day, Marybeth came into Ellen's room and told her she had a surprise. She covered her up with a warm flannel blanket as it was a cool but sunny day. Marybeth wheeled Ellen's bed outside the main door where other staff were waiting. As Ellen sat in her bed, warm and cozy, the staff dumped buckets of colorful leaves they had collected over top of her. She breathed in the smell of the leaves, remembering her days walking in the forest. She lifted her face to feel the fresh fall breeze blowing on her skin. Next, came the pumpkins! Ellen spent an enjoyable hour helping to carve the pumpkins which were later put in a row on a shelf in her room. Then, with tears running down her face, she said, "Enjoying my last autumn was something I never thought I would ever be able to do. Thank you for giving me the chance to live this moment."

Unfinished goals take on a sudden urgency that is not present when people are healthy and think they have all the time in the world. When someone is dying, they realize the window of opportunity is narrower and, due to the burden of their symptoms, they may require the assistance of others to accomplish what is most important to them.

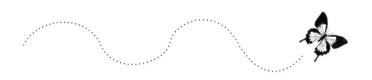

AN ANGEL IN THE MAKING

This is the only story I have included involving a child. I do not have the expertise to care for children who are dying, and I thank those that do. They inspire me to be the best I can be and I keep them in my thoughts and prayers because I believe they are as close to angels as anyone can be.

This story is about a little six-year-old named Carol Ann. She was in the hospital dying of kidney failure and only lived about a week after I met her. Her aunt was her caregiver as her parents had died in a car accident and so, naturally, she was under a great deal of stress and guarded her niece against any talk of death or dying. In fact, she kept telling her that she was looking better. Aunt Shana never left her alone when Marybeth or any other caregiver was in the room to ensure that the conversations with Carol Ann only included the "safe" topics.

As time went on and Shana trusted the staff, she gradually left them alone with her niece for short periods. One day, Shana decided to go for a coffee break while Marybeth bathed Carol Ann. As Marybeth gently washed Carol Ann's thin little arms, Carol Ann asked, "What color of dresses do angels wear?"

Marybeth responded "Well, I believe they wear beautiful white dresses."

Carol Ann's next response brought tears to Marybeth's eyes. She confided, "I want to wear a beautiful white dress when I go to meet the angels, but my auntie doesn't want to talk about that because it makes her too sad. Can I wear a white dress when I go to heaven? Would I look pretty? Would you ask my auntie if she can buy me a white dress?"

Marybeth hugged Carol Ann and told her she would look beautiful in a white dress and that the angels would love to be her friend.

When Carol Ann's aunt returned, Marybeth took her aside and told her what her niece had said. She told Shana that she believed that Carol Ann knew she was going to die and needed to be able to talk about it with the one she loved—her aunt. The most important thing to Carol Ann at that time was to be able to wear a beautiful white dress when she died. Shana sat and cried.

The next day, Carol Ann's aunt arrived with five white dresses for her to try on. The joy on Carol Ann's face would be forever remembered. She tried on each dress, admiring them in the mirror that Marybeth brought into her room. She chose her favourite white dress, and it was draped over the back of her hospital bed for the rest of her stay.

Carol Ann was changed into her beautiful dress before she became unconscious. She truly looked like a little angel. Any parent would be proud to send off their little child to heaven cloaked in angelic beauty.

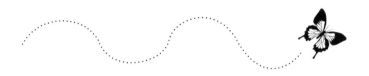

COMFORT IN DEMENTIA

Martha came to us with extensive disease that required total care. She had stopped eating and drinking, was totally bed ridden and was almost comatose. We didn't believe she would survive more than a few days.

Martha not only survived, but she gradually began to improve. The palliative doctor felt it was because of the compassionate care and the good homemade food she was receiving at the hospice. Her cancer tumor was also growing slower than anticipated. Martha went from requiring total feeding to feeding herself. One day Marybeth found her shoveling a pancake into her mouth with her hands, her arms covered in syrup, and the plate stuck to her elbow.

Martha was also diagnosed with end-stage dementia. This diagnosis can present many concerns for a caregiver. Sometimes you have to go along with what your patient is telling you, whether real or perceived as real, so as not to escalate the situation and cause more distress.

One day Martha declared that her pink nightgown was missing. However she hadn't brought a pink nightgown to the hospice, nor did she even own one. She became quite obsessed about whether this precious item had been lost or stolen, and she could not settle.

Marybeth found a new white nightgown that had been donated to the hospice and washed it with a load of the red towels kept on hand for emergencies. The nightgown came out, you guessed it, pink. When Marybeth presented it to Martha, she was overjoyed that it had been found. She wore her pink nightgown every day and eagerly waited for it to be returned to her each laundry day.

As Martha spent hours lying in bed watching people walking by in the hallway, she would play with the edge of her bed sheet, as this gave her comfort. Marybeth brought in a stuffed toy puppy, intending to give it to Martha as a tactile alternative. However, the puppy was accidentally knocked to the ground while Marybeth cleaned Martha's room. Martha called Marybeth over and urgently whispered that she could see a puppy hiding beside the couch and that he looked scared. Marybeth picked up the puppy and handed it to Martha, who began to pet and comfort it. She kept the puppy with her in bed, and they became inseparable. She told everyone the story of how the scared little puppy hiding in the corner had just hopped up on her bed one day and was now hers to keep.

The sensation of touch can be very important to people at the end of life, and also to people who have dementia. It is similar to a child who has a security blanket. Whether it is someone's hand to hold or a lost puppy, it can bring comfort and reassurance.

Mary Gatschene

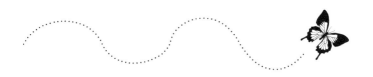

THE LAST BIRTHDAY

Ron was a seventy year-old who was admitted to hospice with end-stage bowel cancer. His wife, Joanne, was his whole life. He received many visitors, but he just wanted his wife by his side, even if she only sat beside him quietly reading.

As Ron got closer to death, he wanted some quality time alone with Joanne. Her birthday was coming up the following week, and this would be the last birthday they would spend together. Marybeth knew how important they were to each other, so she asked Ron if he'd like the staff to arrange a surprise birthday lunch for just the two of them. His eyes opened wide and he said, "You could do that?" He continued that he had wanted to plan something special for his wife's birthday but was too weak and was running out of time.

So on the chosen day, the staff gathered what they needed. Joanne was asked to wait in the lounge as the nurse needed to do an assessment on Ron. The staff then quickly decorated a table in his room using a white sheet as a tablecloth. They arranged flowers in a vase on the table and set out wine glasses filled with ginger ale and cranberry juice. Candles were place on the table and lit. Romantic piano music played on the CD player. A sign was affixed to the door announcing the "Moment in Time" restaurant. Ron was dressed by staff and assisted into a chair.

When everything was ready, Joanne was brought to the room. She was curious about the sign on the door and opened it slowly. Inside, she found Ron with a huge smile on his face, sitting at a table covered with flowers, candles and wine glasses, surrounded by balloons and romantic music. Crying, she hurried over and hugged him, saying, "Ron, I love you."

The hospice staff were also in tears as they took photos of Ron and his wife. The volunteer on duty that day had prepared a special lunch of pasta and salad. For dessert, Marybeth presented chocolate cupcakes, one with a lit birthday candle. Ron and Joanne had an uninterrupted private birthday lunch.

Later, Joanne said it was her best birthday ever and she would cherish the photos. Ron said he couldn't believe the hospice staff would plan all this for someone they hardly knew, and asked how he could repay them. Marybeth replied that the joy on his and his wife's faces was payment enough and that it was an honor to be a part of the celebration.

During his last week of life, Ron told everyone who came to visit him about the best birthday party he ever attended and all the love that surrounded him on that special day.

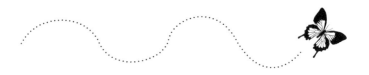

A DRINK (OR TWO) IS
GOOD FOR THE SOUL

Ann enjoyed a drink before bed once in a while—a "bloody Caesar," to be exact. Since coming to the hospice, her appetite had become almost non-existent. She said that nothing tasted good and she just did not feel like eating. Besides, what was the point? She knew she was dying, so why bother? She did, however, have a craving for one last Caesar.

It was discussed with her doctor, and he gave an order that she could have an alcoholic drink once in a while. Each time the doctor visited he said, "Well, have you had your drink yet?" and she replied that she was still waiting for her husband to bring it in.

Finally, one day Bob, her husband, took Marybeth aside and, with a wink, handed her a plastic bag containing a small bottle of vodka. Marybeth put it in the fridge in the medication room to keep it safe.

The next doctor's day, Bob and Marybeth decided that Ann should be sipping her Caesar when the doctor arrived. Marybeth got some celery from the kitchen and mixed the drink, adding some tomato juice and spices that Bob brought in. She draped a towel over her arm, like a waiter, and knocked on Ann's door. She announced to Ann that she was bringing her the drink she'd ordered from the bar. Ann laughed and clapped her hands. She took a sip and smiled. Marybeth told her that the doctor should be arriving shortly.

That morning the doctor was late. By the time he made rounds, he found Ann sitting in bed with an empty glass and rosy red cheeks. All that was left was a piece of soggy celery. Ann had gotten tired of waiting for him, so she drank the whole glass. She told the doctor that next time she might even share some with him—as long as he was on time for "happy hour."

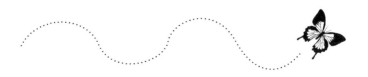

THE POWER OF MUSIC

Hannah loved music and had spent many years singing in a choir and playing the guitar. When Marybeth invited her to the lounge one evening to listen to her playing the piano, Hannah agreed with a smile on her face. She was wheeled to the lounge in her bed, excited about going to the "concert." At first there were no other residents in the lounge, and Hannah was impressed that she was being given a "private" concert. She sang along to the songs and hummed when she didn't know the words.

After an hour, Hannah had fallen asleep, but awoke as she was being wheeled back to her room. She asked Marybeth if there was a concert every Sunday and, if so, how could she sign up to attend?

The next day, Marybeth heard singing coming from Hannah's room. Knocking on the door, she entered to find Hannah sitting in bed with one hand scrolling through song lyrics on her laptop screen, and the other hand holding her hairbrush to her mouth as a microphone. She grinned at Marybeth and handed her the hairbrush. Marybeth joined in and as more staff arrived they too sang in harmony. After twenty minutes of singing, with a hoarse voice and a smile, Hannah leaned back on her pillows and said, "Thank you all for attending my concert."

Music has proven to be a great stress reliever and to give a great deal of comfort to many people who are dying. Some residents like to hum or sing at our "concerts" and some just like to listen. Whether they are tone deaf or have the voice of an angel, everyone is allowed to join in. Even when they are not responding, residents will often settle and become less agitated and restless when caregivers turn on some soft, quiet music or family members sit by their side holding their hand and singing to them. Remember, hearing is one of the last senses to leave us. It's possible to purchase CDs of instrumental music played at a slower speed to resemble the slowing beat of your heart for people who are nearing death. A music therapist once commented that several times when she was singing by herself to residents, they told her they loved the "harmony" they heard, even though there was nobody else in the room. Perhaps they heard angels singing along.

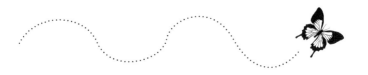

I'M STILL IN CHARGE

I will never forget one of the first times I witnessed a conversation between a palliative doctor and her patient. I was new to the field of palliative care and had much to learn. I was caring for Jill in the hospital. She was thirty-five years old and dying of cancer. She was losing her independence and she now required assistance to get out of bed, to bathe and to feed herself. Many people at the end of life still want to maintain their independence and make their own decisions regarding their care. As they deteriorate physically, they must depend on others to care for them. As long as they are competent to make decisions about their goals of care they should be encouraged to do so. The discussion I witnessed was both compassionate and courageous.

I, as Jill's caregiver, was not comfortable discussing the intimate details regarding the subject of dying. This compassionate doctor sat beside Jill and told her they were going to discuss Jill's death and what that would look like and what Jill was hoping for. I remember thinking "hoping for?" What was there to hope for—she was dying and there was nothing we could do about it.

They discussed whether Jill wanted to be awake and alert or whether she wanted to be more sedate and not as aware. Jill spoke of a repeating dream she was having where she saw a partially open door with bright light shining from the other side. Her doctor asked her what she thought of that. Jill stated that it was pulling her closer and she wanted to go through the door. The doctor told her that if that was her wish, she should go through the door. I could not believe the openness and comfort that came through in their conversation. After more discussion, Jill decided she wanted to be awake and alert to say goodbye to her family and friends, even though it meant she would be in more pain. She wanted to take less pain medication so her mind would be clearer. Once she had said goodbye she wanted her medication increased so she was sedate and pain-free.

Jill thanked the doctor for giving her the power to be in charge of her life and for caring about her wishes. She stated that her family and friends did not want to talk about her death and how she saw it happening, which caused her further distress.

We often don't know what to say to those who are dying, and sometimes the most important way to help is to just listen and let them control where the conversation leads them. People have the right to express their wishes and have us follow through with them even if they don't correspond to our wishes for them.

This experience has taught me what many people at the end of life actually "hope" for. They hope for a pain-free death, a death with a loved one holding their hand, to be unconscious and unaware when dying, to be remembered and to have made a difference in someone's life, for a special visit from someone they have not seen for a long time, for forgiveness, to be alone and not have their family watch them die, to achieve that one last item on their "bucket list."

One of our roles as caregivers is to help people in our care to refocus their hopes onto things than can be realistically achieved. Have you ever gone on a journey without being prepared? People in our care are embarking on their last journey and they also want to be prepared. We need to have the courage to discuss openly and comfortably what they wish for and keep them involved in treatment and care decisions.

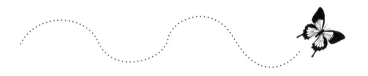

COMPASSION LONG DISTANCE

My husband had an aunt, Helen, who lived in California. She became ill and was not able to get out of bed. She had caregivers around the clock. Helen had enjoyed visiting her only sister in Canada every year, but now she hadn't seen her in almost two years.

I called Helen one day to tell her that my husband and I were bringing my mother-in-law to visit her in California. She said, "That will happen when hell freezes over. I will believe it when I see her walk in the door." She couldn't imagine her elderly sister travelling such a distance just to see her.

I asked her if there was anything she needed, and she replied that she wanted to be able to get out of bed. Her caregivers told her this was not possible because she could not stand, but they had never tried to get her up.

When I called her the week before our trip, she instructed her caregivers to get the house in order. She did not want her cherished Christmas decorations put away because she wanted us to see the collection of animated dolls she had spent years collecting.

A few days before we left, I called to get an update on Helen's condition. I spoke with the visiting nurse who said that the doctor did not know if she would live long enough to see us. Helen wanted so desperately to see her sister that I just knew she would stay alive to have one final visit.

There were tears of joy when we arrived, and the sisters gave each other a big hug. As Helen was still able to eat, we told her that we would get her lunch from wherever she wanted, thinking we would have a meal from some awesome restaurant that we did not have in Canada. But she wanted a Big Mac from McDonalds—so that is what we got.

As soon as lunch was finished, Aunt Helen said, "Okay, when can I get up?" We decided to wait until the next day, as we planned a special dinner for her. We had invited her two best friends to join us for dinner, one of whom was in her 90s. We had ordered a special cake decorated with the words "good friends" and were going to bring in Chinese food (her favourite).

The next morning, I asked her, "If you could have one wish today, what would it be?" She said she would love to go into each room in her house, as she hadn't been in any room other than where she was now in months.

We had bought her some new nightgowns and had them altered so they had snaps in the back and were easy to put on. She chose her favourite one to wear for her dinner party.

We were able to get her up from her bed with the use of a transfer disk and with her hanging on to me for dear life. She hadn't been out of bed for over a month and was terrified of falling. We successfully got her comfortable in her wheelchair.

She looked like a queen in her new nightgown, wrapped in a blanket, sitting up in her chair. We wheeled her into each room of her house where she just sat and looked around. Afterwards, we had a great meal together with her friends.

After we got her back to bed, she leaned over to my husband and said, "Thank you for bringing my sister to me."

We spent wonderful days visiting her, then continued on to San Francisco with the promise that we would see her again in five days when we returned.

On our drive back we phoned ahead to let her know we were arriving later in the day. We were told she had become very confused and agitated, and the doctor had to be called. When we arrived, she had deteriorated and was barely responding. We were due to return home the next day and were not able to change our plans. We hugged her and told her we loved her. We left with a sadness in our hearts because we knew we were saying goodbye forever.

We got a call forty-eight hours after we returned home to say that she had died. It had been a very peaceful death. We were grateful that we had some great moments that mattered to all of us and we brought her some laughter, love and compassion even for a short time.

As people get closer to dying, they often get a last burst of energy to wait for that special moment in time, that chance to say goodbye to a special person, that special occasion coming up—and somehow they are given the strength to survive until that goal is accomplished. We were so thankful that Helen found that strength and that we made the trip to bring her family to her.

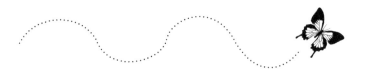

LAST CANADA DAY
CELEBRATION

This was going to be the last Canada Day cel-
ebrated by our current residents, so the hospice
staff planned a barbeque for July 1. Both residents
and their families joined in the celebration in the
outside sitting area, which was decorated with
Canadian flags and streamers. The staff barbequed
chicken, provided potato salad and served ice cream
for dessert. Some residents were only able to take
one bite of their chicken or have one teaspoon of ice
cream, as it took a great deal of energy to do even
that, but all the residents wanted to participate.
Everyone sang "Oh Canada."

Imagine the sight! Hospital beds sitting on patio
stones, holding residents wrapped in warm blankets because they felt chilly even on a hot summer
evening. Under those warm blankets were pain
pumps, drainage bags and oxygen tubing, but the
beds had one thing in common: All the occupants

had smiles on their face— proud Canadians celebrating one last time with glowing hearts in the land they call home.

The residents all shared the experience of being surrounded by love and compassion. The family members all shared a bonding of new friendships with people coping together during a difficult time. Isn't this what being Canadian is all about? We are fighting our battles together with the strength of other Canadians supporting us, whether the enemy comes from inside us as a cancerous tumor or from some external source.

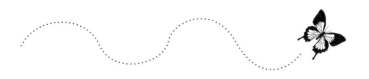

WHY AM I STILL ALIVE?

I cared for a very insightful man named Jim who had a terminal disease and was restricted to a wheelchair and only able to transfer with assistance. He was not able to speak, so he used a wipe-off board to communicate. He lived with his daughter, who was his main caregiver. He also had a personal support worker who lived in the basement apartment of his house and assisted him daily with morning care.

At the end of every visit I would ask Jim if he had any questions for me, and every time he would ask the same question—"Why am I still alive? I am no good to anyone." He would have a distressed look on his face as he struggled for an answer. I decided I needed to come up with one that would ease his mind and preserve his sense of worth.

At our next visit I asked that same question, and once again he gave me the same response. But this time I had a reply. "Jim, I have been thinking about the answer to that question, and I think the reason you are still alive is because you are still needed. What if you are not alive for you, but for your daughter? What if your daughter is going to face something in her life where she will need a great deal of strength and compassion to survive? By having had the opportunity to care for you, she will have learned compassion and gained strength to cope with whatever she will encounter. It will be because of you that she will have the skills to overcome any stressful situation in her life. That will be your legacy to her."

Jim sat there deep in thought and then wrote, "I never thought about it like that." Jim never asked the question again, and seemed more at peace and content.

I don't claim to know the answer to his question, but hopefully offered him an answer that allowed him to keep his dignity and show him that he still had something to give—he was needed and did indeed make a difference in someone else's life.

People need to feel they are worth something and still have something to give, especially when facing life-limiting illnesses. People who are struggling with health challenges are better able to cope when they find value in their lives. We need to help them find that internal sense of comfort and peace.

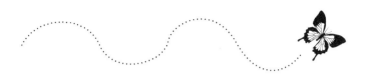

CANDLES FOR EVERYONE

Many hospices have rituals they follow when a resident dies. At one hospice, they have a special blanket to cover the resident on the stretcher when the funeral home arrives. Another hospice has a designated table where a lighted candle is placed and burns in memory of the resident after they have died. Many hospices have a procession from the resident's room out to the funeral vehicle with a family member carrying a lighted candle at the head of the procession. These rituals are very beautiful and respectful of the person who has died.

One morning the staff at a hospice, which followed a ritual with lighted candles, started their shift with one candle burning for a resident who had died overnight. Later that morning, Marybeth noticed that there were three candles burning. She was shocked, as she had just had a break with the other team members and nobody had reported any other deaths that day.

A man was standing in front of the table with the candles. As Marybeth approached him, he said, "Oh, I think this is wonderful how people can come and light a candle here. I lit one for my mom and one for my dad."

Marybeth gently explained to him the purpose of the candles. He apologized for lighting them and, after saying a prayer for his parents, he smiled and blew out the candles.

I have seen family members stop on their way out the door and just stand in front of the candle burning for their loved one, close their eyes or touch the container holding the candle, perhaps saying a last farewell to them. We respect all our residents, and this candle ritual is our way of saying thank you to them for giving us the opportunity to have been a part of their lives.

LIFE'S JOURNEY

Palliative care --an approach that improves the quality of life of person and their families facing the issues associated with life-threatening illness------- "to cloak"

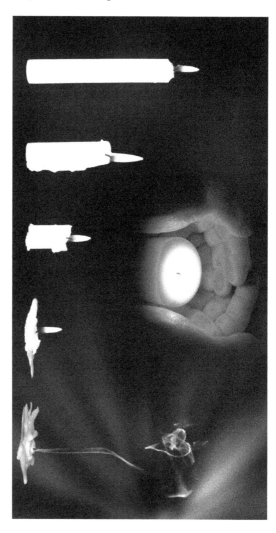

We are like a candle whose flame is burning with life

Our flame changes and moulds us through our life's journey

When our goals are reached it burns stronger and brighter.

During times of stress our flame can dim and then...

When our flame can no longer burn and we are at the end of life, we reach out to our circle of care, to be cloaked in compassion

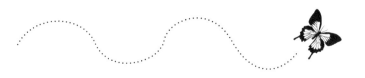

HAND IN HAND

When Cindy came to our hospice she had to leave her husband at home alone and she missed him dearly. He was not well, but wasn't diagnosed with a life-threatening illness so he did not qualify to be admitted to the hospice along with her. His children brought him to visit whenever they could, and Cindy would sit with him, holding his hand. He called her every morning, and she made sure she was sitting by the phone to take the call.

One day Cindy came slowly down the hallway with her walker, looking distressed and very upset. She sat in her favourite chair facing the window, breathing heavily and crying. When Marybeth hurried over, Cindy sobbed that her husband was not well and had been admitted to the hospital. He was going to be okay, but could not go home. Cindy could speak with him on the phone, she explained, "But he is there, and I am here, and we are both alone."

Marybeth held her hand, and together they prayed for her husband and for the nursing staff who would be caring for him. Cindy thanked Marybeth for the beautiful prayer and for caring and told her the story of her life with her husband. "Do you know that this summer we will celebrate our sixty-fourth wedding anniversary?" she asked. Cindy said she knew time was running out for both of them, and she wished they could be together when they died.

One week later her husband was discharged from the hospital, and the family brought him to visit Cindy. She sat on the couch by the front window holding hands with him and smiling. She said "I am so happy. My husband came to see me." Marybeth hoped they could be together when the time came for Cindy to die, and promised her she would do whatever she could to make that happen.

Cindy deteriorated more quickly than expected. Her family was called in to be with her as she was dying. A bed was set up beside Cindy, and her husband slept beside her on her last night. She died peacefully with loved ones by her side.

Sometimes living every moment can be as simple as just sitting and talking to a resident, allowing them to tell their story or to voice their concerns.

Cindy became very close to her caregivers and trusted them with her life. She often told the doctor, "They are so good to me. They always know what I like and they listen to me." We are not able to solve every issue, but we can listen with compassion and offer emotional comfort.

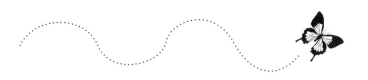

DANNY BOY

Ann was one of the first residents in a newly-opened hospice. She was there for several months and she had unending patience with the staff during their growing pains. She had a great sense of humor and shared many laughs with her care team. Ann accepted her fate in life and just lived one day at a time. Her husband, Bob, was very much in love with her and was at her side caring for her as much as he was able to. He came in every day, and the hospice became his second home.

Ann loved music. Her favourite song was "Danny Boy." She and Bob had decided many years ago that when one of them died, the other would play that song at the funeral as a reminder that they would be waiting for their loved one.

Because music can be a great therapy to provide comfort in times of stress, Marybeth would some-times play the piano for the residents. They would have concerts in the lounge, sitting by the fireplace on a quiet day, humming along to the songs. One day, Bob asked Marybeth if she could play "Danny Boy," but she did not have the music. Several days later, as Bob was leaving the hospice, Marybeth called him over to the piano and began to play "Danny Boy." As she played, he cried and told of the promise he and his wife had made to each other.

The next evening, Marybeth asked Ann if she and her visiting daughter would like a private piano concert in the lounge. Ann happily agreed, saying she felt like a kid sneaking out because she would normally be getting ready for bed at this time of night. Marybeth told Ann that she had a special song for her and began to play "Danny Boy." Ann and her daughter sang along, the words having long ago been memorized, while tears rolled down their faces.

The next day, Ann phoned Bob first thing in the morning to tell him of the private concert she attended late at night and how much it meant to her. Music can evoke many emotions and can bring us peace in difficult times. It allows us to recall memories from our past and create new memories for our future.

Ann and Bob's family and friends were amazed at the thoughtfulness the staff showed to them at the hospice and how they created special moments in such a loving manner. Bob was so appreciative of the care they both received that even after Ann died he came to visit the staff and let them know how he was managing at home without his wife. He gave everyone he knew a hug. The song "Danny Boy" will always remind me of Ann and Bob and their heartfelt promise to each other.

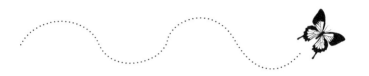

THE BEST TRIP EVER

Caitlin was a beautiful, fun-loving resident who stayed at our hospice for about four months. She rarely had any complaints and did not like to "bother" the staff. She was shy and had a definite serenity about her. She valued her friends and family and enjoyed their visits. We learned so much from her about how to cherish life and take one day at a time.

Day after day went by and she still had a smile and a kind word for everyone. Her husband had a difficult time watching her becoming more fatigued and losing so much weight. The hospice staff supported him during the more difficult days, as he felt so helpless.

Caitlin decided to write her legacy with assistance from a dignity therapy staff member. She agreed to let Marybeth read it. She wrote that her only big regret was never having had the opportunity to go on a cruise to Amsterdam and Austria because she could not afford it and did not have the time. Now, of course, it was too late.

Marybeth thought: if Caitlin could not go on a cruise, could the staff bring a cruise to Caitlin? She and her co-workers began to plan. Local travel agents were contacted and they provided pictures, magazines and videos about cruises in Europe. A grocery store donated a cheese tray, fruit tray and dessert tray for the surprise buffet. Drinks, chips (one of Caitlin's favorite foods), vegetables and other food items were donated by staff members. One staff member made an ice sculpture. Permission was given for Caitlin, her spouse and friends to have an alcoholic beverage (Bailey's was Caitlin's favorite). One staff member added the sound of a cruise ship horn to her cell phone to play as the "ship" was leaving. Boarding passes for a "virtual cruiseline" were printed for Caitlin and her travel group. A CD of ocean wave sounds was set up in her room. A gift bag with items from Europe (soap, shampoo, chocolate, cookies, tea) was prepared. One staff member rehearsed a song and dance show for the cruise's entertainment component. A PowerPoint presentation was set up in Caitlin's room to display photos and information about each European town visited on this cruise. Balloons were donated by a local store to decorate her room. Many staff members who were not on duty that day came to help and to act as the other passengers on the cruise ship. Her spouse and friends knew about the plans, but it was to be a surprise for Caitlin.

On the day of the cruise, Caitlin's friend and spouse came to visit and took her to the lounge for a "change of scenery." The moment she left her room, the team got to work decorating her "suite" with travel posters and a porthole so she could imagine looking out at the ocean. Other staff transformed the sun room into a ship's buffet.

When everything was ready, Marybeth went to get Caitlin. She handed her the boarding pass in an envelope, stating that it had been dropped off at the front desk. Caitlin opened it, read the boarding pass, and sighed, "That would be nice." Her husband and friend showed her that they had also received boarding passes. Marybeth urged them to go quickly because the ship was boarding at 1 p.m. and it was almost that time.

As Marybeth wheeled a confused Caitlin down to the "cruise ship," they could hear the ship's horn sounding. Caitlin was astonished at the transformed room and the waiting staff. The look on her face said it all. She was handed a glass of Bailey's, a sunhat was placed on her head and she was given flowers. Then everyone "cruised" through Europe along with the PowerPoint presentation.

When the cruise was over, Marybeth said, "I don't know about the rest of you, but I am hungry. Don't they have a buffet on this cruise?" Caitlin was then wheeled into the sun room for the buffet, which she greatly enjoyed, especially the chips and desserts. The entertainment came next, receiving great applause from Caitlin and her fellow "passengers." She was then presented with a gift bag. Caitlin sat there with tears in her eyes and kept repeating, "I can't believe this."

The staff thought Caitlin would be exhausted by now and would want to go to bed to rest, but they were wrong. She was having too much fun. She lounged in her wheelchair and was given a foot soak and massage while soft music and the sound of waves played in the background. A diffuser with essential oils enhanced the relaxed and calming atmosphere.

When Caitlin was finally ready for bed, she cried and told Marybeth, "It was the best trip I have ever been on. Thank you."

Marybeth replied, "You are very special to us, and we wanted to do something special for you."

That is a trip we will never forget. It not only made a special memory for Caitlin and her family, but it also brought our staff together and made everyone feel great! Caitlin had never allowed pictures to be taken of her in her last few months, but she agreed to have some taken of her cruise. They were put in a photo album, and Caitlin delighted in showing them to all her visitors. She was often observed sitting in bed, looking at them over and over again.

There was not a dry eye on the best cruise ever that day.

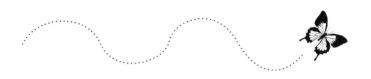

A GIFT TO CHERISH—
FROM MOTHER TO SON

Laura came to our hospice for a tour two days before being admitted. Her husband, Scott, and twelve-year-old son, Ryan, were with her as she wanted to assure herself that they would be comfortable and supportive in her choice of her final "home." She did not want to die at home and leave that memory for her son to live with for the rest of his life.

Laura wanted to leave a part of herself with her son so he would always remember her and be comforted in times of stress. It had to be a gift that would nourish his spirit as he grew into adulthood, something that would capture the essence of her. Due to the spread of her cancer, she experienced pain and fatigue and did not have the energy to coordinate and follow through with her plan. Marybeth discussed an idea with Laura regarding a gift for her son that would bond them together;

a moment in time that he could cherish. Laura cried tears of relief as they began to plan for that special moment.

One week later Ryan was visiting, and Marybeth asked him if he wanted to work on a project with his mom. She brought out some plaster in a foil pan, added some water, and then they got messy. Laura made an imprint in the plaster with her hand, and Ryan did the same, their thumbs touching to form the shape of a heart. They carved the date beneath their handprint and placed glass stones inside the heart. Ryan had a great time with his mom. They both had plaster on their hands, arms and shirts and on Laura's bed—it really was messy!

Marybeth explained to Ryan that if he was ever feeling sad he could put his hand in the imprint of his mom's hand and feel her love and strength; that every wrinkle and vein in the handprint belonged only to his mom, as no two are the same. She told him it was an amazing gift from his mom and that he would have a part of her forever.

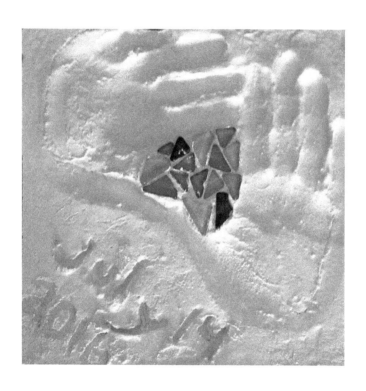

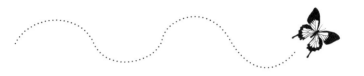

THE FINAL GRADUATION

We admitted a young forty-four-year-old resident, Erin, who had been fighting cancer for three years. It had now spread to several main organs, and she knew she was losing the fight. She had a twelve-year-old son, Ryan, with whom she had a very special relationship. Ryan understood why his mom had been admitted and he had been given a tour of the hospice prior to her accepting the bed. He stated that he thought his mom would be "safe" at the hospice and he would enjoy the video games in the children's room and all the cookies set out for family to enjoy when he visited her.

Erin knew that her son was putting on a brave face, but he was afraid of her dying. She cried as she told Marybeth that the night before, her son had slept in her hospital bed at home because he missed her. She also told Marybeth that she wished she could die quickly so as not to put Ryan through any more grief.

While she was in hospice, Erin's son graduated from grade six. She was planning to go to his graduation ceremony the next day. Afterwards, her husband would bring Ryan, his friend and several others to the hospice where they would order in dinner together. They had reserved the sunroom.

Marybeth asked Erin if the staff could decorate the sunroom for the party. She loved that idea. Marybeth then asked Erin if they had a graduation cake. Erin stated that she hadn't had the time or energy to arrange it, and did not want to bother her husband. Marybeth asked her permission for the staff to bring in a cake. Erin got tears in her eyes and said it would be a wonderful surprise for her son.

Marybeth was able to get a graduation cake donated from a local grocery store. The staff at the hospice brought in decorations, balloons and bowls of gummy worms and jelly beans. While Erin was at Ryan's graduation, the sunroom was decorated, and a banner was placed above the doorway. The staff signed a graduation poster with congratulatory messages and blessings for the future for Erin's son.

Erin felt proud showing her visitors the "party room" decorated for this special day. Ryan and his friend grinned as their hands dug into the bowls of candy (the gummy worms were a big hit with the boys).

Later, Erin told Marybeth that the celebration was perfect. She thanked the staff for making this moment so special, as this would be the final graduation she would share with her son.

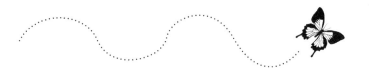

THE "TIME-OUT" CLASS

Jemma had been diagnosed with end-stage lung cancer. She was not a candidate for chemotherapy, as the cancer was too advanced. She was an active woman and struggled with having to slow down due to her breathlessness.

When she was admitted to hospice she became depressed and found the days very long. Marybeth invited Jemma to join the art class, where she could pass the time painting on canvas. She replied that the only thing she had ever painted was a bedroom for her daughter— there was more paint on herself than on the wall. She was sure she did not have the talent to paint an actual picture. Marybeth replied that it did not require talent because everyone painted from the heart. No painting was of lesser quality, because it was as individual as the painter. Besides, she did not have to exert herself physically while painting, so her breathing would not be laboured. Marybeth told her there was only one rule in the class—everyone had to talk about something cheerful. Jemma decided to give it a try.

Jemma had some of her best moments in that class. She felt free to enjoy the life around her. She sat at a table with several other residents, painting and discussing memories from their pasts with laughter, teasing and just great camaraderie— with no talk of disease and illness. The participants found the class very refreshing; it took them away from their world of stress for a well-needed "time-out."

As it turned out, Jemma did indeed have talent. Her paintings were admired by many staff and visitors. She described one of her paintings of a cottage. Her parents had taken her there every summer. Jemma would often go to play along the beach and pick rocks or feed the ducks. This painting represented a special time in her life. She felt honoured to present Marybeth with her work of art, as she no longer had any family to appreciate it. To this day, the painting hangs in Marybeth's house and she is amazed at the hidden talent that was set free during a time of stress and illness.

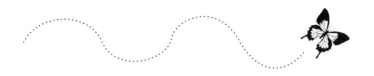

THE LAST SURPRISE

I remember caring for Doug, a very proud, private gentleman in the community who was diagnosed with cancer. He never complained or let his wife know how unwell he was feeling. His wife was a courageous, strong woman and remained by his side through his gradual decline, caring for him with loving hands and always being his advocate.

As Doug became weaker and more fatigued, he decided he wanted to have one more special night out with his wife. When she came home from running errands one day, he told her to get dressed up, as they were going out. He wouldn't tell her where they were going—only that she needed to look "fancy."

Doug insisted on driving and, to her surprise, drove for an hour into Toronto, to an upscale restaurant where he had made dinner reservations.

Even though he had not been eating well lately, he was able to enjoy his entire dinner.

After dinner, they went for a walk. His wife could see he was fatigued and somewhat short of breath, but he assured her he was fine and just needed to go slowly. As they walked by a theater, Doug suggested, "Let's go in and see what is playing here." When they entered, he reached into his pocket and pulled out two tickets to the show, "Dixieland Jazz" (from New Orleans). Although Doug had to stand outside the theatre towards the end of the show due to the pain in his leg, he insisted that they stay for the entire performance.

They had a wonderful evening. After the show, as they walked to their car in the cold winter rain, Doug's wife removed her coat and covered his head to keep him dry. She drove home as he sat beside her, very fatigued but grateful that he was able to accomplish his goal and have a memorable night out.

I always stress the importance of making moments matter, and this gentleman, even though he was not well, still found the strength to do something that was obviously very important to him. He took a chance and persevered through his pain and fatigue, hoping he would be well enough for this special moment to share with his wife. She now has this lasting memory to cherish because she knows what it took for him to plan and follow through with giving her this last gift to show his love.

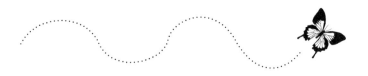

MAKE IT A SUGAR SHACK

Brian lived in a small cottage in the country. He became ill and was diagnosed with stage-four cancer. He had past medical training, so he understood his disease process very well and knew what would likely transpire in the weeks ahead. He found the days long and would often sit on his front porch and watch the world go by. Marybeth would often sit with him and share a cup of tea on her many visits as his palliative nurse.

One day, Brian watched some men hauling construction supplies across the road at the neighbor's house. As they started building, he and Marybeth wondered what was being erected. Brian fancifully hoped it was a sugar shack (it was actually a market stall). He told Marybeth how he loved to eat pancakes with real maple syrup poured over top.

When the building was almost finished, Marybeth decided to surprise Brian by creating a sugar shack. On the weekend, when the construction team was not working, Marybeth set up a table and chairs in front of the new building after getting permission from the owner. Some of her co-workers brought pancakes and a fresh bottle of maple syrup from a nearby sugar bush. They taped a "Sugar Shack" sign to the building. Marybeth had arranged for Brian's friend to take him for a walk outside in his wheelchair and bring him over to the new building.

When they arrived at the front of the building, Marybeth waved and called out, "Come and have a treat at the Sugar Shack."

Brian had a grin on his face and when he was offered some pancakes with fresh maple syrup on top he said, "This brings back some awesome memories of helping my dad in the sugar bush."

Brian and his friends spent a lovely afternoon together enjoying their special treat.

A few weeks later, Brian told Marybeth that the sugar shack was his best memory since he became ill. He said it was magical how it appeared so suddenly one day, just when he needed a special moment to boost his spirits.

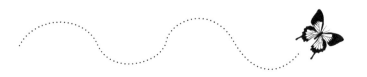

A FRIEND IN MY ROOM

Many people who come from home and have been surrounded by family members twenty-four hours a day have a difficult time being alone once they come to hospice. Family members are often exhausted from caring for their loved one, and the lack of sleep eventually catches up to them. Once their loved one is admitted to hospice, it is important for family members to get rested so they can be re-energized for the tough road ahead.

If there is an unlimited supply of family members to take turns staying overnight with their loved one, that is ideal. However, few people have so many care-givers. An elderly lady, Joan, who came from a small family, was admitted to hospice. When her family left to go home at night, she would cry and call out for them to sit with her as she did not want to be alone. She was also somewhat confused and her eyesight was poor so she felt even more uncomfortable at night.

One night, after hearing the elderly resident calling out and crying, Marybeth volunteered to sit with Joan for a while so the staff could finish their night work. She knew that there was a first-aid mannequin stored in a closet on the second floor of the hospice, so she brought the mannequin, propped up in a wheelchair, into Joan's room with her. Joan, on seeing the "person" in the wheelchair, asked who she was. Marybeth replied, "Oh this is Alice. She is my helper. She will just sit in the corner out of the way, and I will stay with you for a while so you are not alone." Joan kept periodically looking at "Alice" and, after about fifteen minutes, commented, "She doesn't say much, does she!" Once Joan finally fell asleep, Marybeth quietly exited the room.

The next morning, the night shift took "Alice" back to her closet. When Marybeth came to work, she learned that Joan had slept well the previous night. Joan told the staff that whenever she woke up she saw "Alice" snoozing or quietly watching over her.

When Joan's family asked about the mysterious "Alice", Marybeth apologized for the deceit as she explained. The family hopefully asked, "Can you put the mannequin there again tonight? Maybe she will sleep again." Marybeth agreed. In fact, Joan requested that her friend "Alice" stay with her every night as she did not bother her and was a comforting presence whenever she woke.

And so for the next week "Alice" spent her nights sitting in the wheelchair in the corner of Joan's room and her days in the closet, Joan slept well as she did not feel alone, and Joan's family slept well at home. After one week they were rested enough to start again staying with Joan at night. Joan occasionally wondered where her friend "Alice" had gone and assumed she must be keeping someone else company at night so they would not be alone.

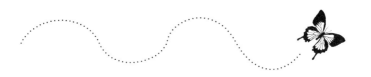

A GIFT TO TAKE TO HEAVEN

I remember when my grandmother died. She was a very special person in my life. Toward the end of her life, my mom cared for her in our house, as it was Grandma's wish to die at home with family by her side. My children were nine and twelve at the time. They were very close to Nana and enjoyed visiting her; she loved to have children around her. You could see the joy in her face as she watched them play. (When my son was around five years old, he would walk around the house with her cane, which was taller than he was, and she found it very amusing.) She always gave the greatest hugs—to children and adults alike. After every visit, she would say, "Next time, stay longer."

When I look back at the time before her death, I recall the night I sat behind her in the bed, holding her as she bolted up and then threw herself back in a delirious state. At that time, I knew very little about end-of-life care and signs of impending death. I did, however, realize that she did not have a great deal of time left to live.

I thought about how my children would react to her death. They were not able to be there during her final few days, so they didn't have a chance to experience their last special moments with her. They needed to be able to say goodbye to Nana in their own way. After some discussion, my children thought they would like to write a note for Nana to take on her journey to Heaven in case she missed them.

We wanted to include our children in the family gathering that would take place so they could understand the importance of such a ritual in our family. My nephew was four years old at the time, and his father explained to him in the simplest way he could that after the funeral they would bury Nana in the ground. My nephew stared up at his dad with a look of wonder on his face, his little nose all scrunched up, and said, "And then another Nana will grow?" (He remembered planting seeds in the ground in the spring and watching them grow). Isn't it amazing what goes through the minds of children and what healing children can bring to us?

Children experience death and grieve differently than adults, depending on their stage of development. It is important not to push our children away in times of grief. They need to feel supported and included in any rituals or customs. They need to understand that it is okay to cry if they are sad and to know that with time there is healing. Including children in these life events will expose them to something we all will experience—the death of a loved one. By doing so, we have the chance to teach them about death in a safe and supported environment, which will aid in their growth and development towards adulthood. These are the poems that my children wrote to their nana.

Dear Nana,

We all loved you,
We didn't want you to die,
We cared about you when
you were in the hospital,
You were kind to your
Great Grandchildren and
loved them.

I love you Nana

Love,
Sarah

It's Not
Over
You brighten up a gloomy day
"You always used to say
"I love my life"
You'd always smile
Your smile was as big as a mile
So hey
You know that we love you
and we miss you too
We will always have a
Place for you in our hearts
We're always learning something
new from you
Good bye my friend it's not
the end
Rest in Pence
We know you can

From Scott

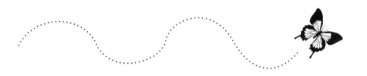

GERRY'S STORY

Gerry was a kind-hearted gentleman who developed a very aggressive type of cancer—a sarcoma. He had tumors on his head that grew rapidly even while he was undergoing fifty-five radiation treatments. The twenty-six tumors required daily dressing changes. He was a stoic man and did not like to complain of pain. Gerry was my father-in-law.

I accompanied Gerry to all his appointments to help him understand the journey he was on. He depended on me to be his advocate. One day after an appointment, I heard someone calling, "Florence! Florence!" down the hall behind us. We continued walking, but the insistent voice repeated the call. I turned to see Gerry's nurse hurrying down the hall to speak with us. She became confused when I told her my name was Mary, not Florence. Gerry, with a grin, admitted that he always referred to me as Florence— his own personal Florence Nightingale.

As his cancer rapidly spread, Gerry was reluctant to take his pain medication, as he did not want to become confused. One day I was sitting beside him as he gently stroked the armrest of his chair. When I asked what he was doing, he replied, "I am petting the dog." There were a few seconds of silence, then he added, "I don't have a dog, do I?"

I replied, "No, but you can pet the chair all you want." He grinned. Shortly after, his pain medication was changed, and his confusion was much improved. Thank goodness the palliative doctor has a variety of opioids to choose from.

As Gerry's journey continued in a downward spiral, we would often discuss the topics of death and dying. I prepared a presentation of his life to be shown at his memorial service and asked him if he wanted to view it, as it would be his legacy to show others all he had accomplished. We watched it together, both of us crying. At the end, I asked him what he thought. He stated, "I don't like the picture of me with the hat on. I want a different picture." We hugged, and I chose another picture with his approval. He told me he was not afraid to die, just afraid of how it would happen. I assured him I would be there to make sure his symptoms were managed, as he was the decision maker of his care.

As he became weaker, he lost his voice and was only able to whisper. He was concerned that he would not be heard if he needed help. I remember sitting in the next room when he called for help. When I got to his bedside, Gerry asked me where I had been as I took too long. He asked his wife to bring his small cow bell and tape it to his bedside so he could ring for me. Watching from the next room, I saw his thin arm reaching for the bell, so I walked over just as he rang it. He looked up at me, startled, and smiled. "Boy, that was fast!" he said.

Later, as he lay in the hospital bed, he said to me with tears in his eyes, "I'm dying, aren't I?" I asked him if he believed he was dying, and he stated "Yes, and I hope I go tonight." He was going to be admitted to the local hospice the next day. He wanted to die at home but, because of the fear that he would have difficulty breathing due to a tumor on his neck, he agreed that he could be better managed at the hospice.

I stayed by his side for the next twenty-four hours of his life. Gerry got his wish, as he did die that night. His breathing stabilized, and he had a very peaceful death with family by his side. We think of him every day and are thankful for the wonderful care and compassion shown to him by all members of his palliative team.

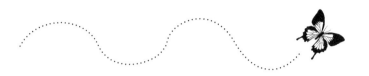

FROM THE AUTHOR:

I hope these stories have inspired people reading them to create those special moments in the lives of their loved ones, to encourage them to live every moment. For those who have identified with the caregiver from their own experiences, I applaud your strength and compassion, because it is a difficult role. We are all important in this journey called life and one day we must all face death. We all wish for a death with dignity and comfort.

The following poem is a favourite of mine. After I read it for the first time, I was left with a feeling of hope and a sense of tranquility. I hope it does the same for all who read it. Oh, and I hope you like the picture. It is my first painting. I think I better stick to nursing, but it does come from the heart

I am standing upon the seashore. A ship at my side spreads her white sails to the morning breeze and starts for the blue ocean. She is an object of beauty and strength. I stand and watch her until at length she hangs like a speck of white cloud just where the sea and sky come to mingle with each other.

When someone at my side says:
"There, she is gone!"

"Gone where?"

"Gone from my sight. That is all." She is just as large in mast and hull and spar as she was when she left my side and she is just as able to bear her load of living freight to her destined port. Her diminished size is in me, not in her.

And just at the moment when someone at my side says, "there, she is gone!" there are other eyes watching her coming, and other voices ready to take up the glad shout:

"Here she comes!" And that is dying...

Death comes in its own time, in its own way. Death is as unique as the individual experiencing it.

By Henry Van Dyke

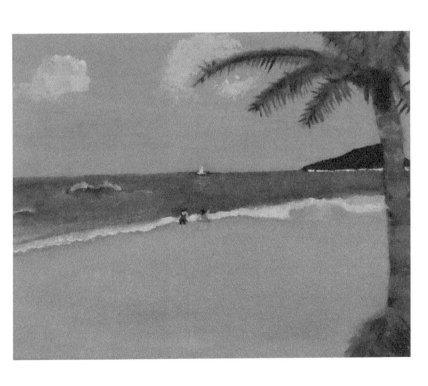

Mary Gatschene

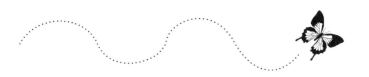

ABOUT THE AUTHOR

Ever since she was a little girl, Mary Gatschene knew she wanted to be a nurse. She studied nursing at a College in Ontario and graduated as a Registered Nurse. She has worked in nursing for over thirty years and in multiple roles including hospital nursing, emergency travel repatriation services, community nursing, health training and as an educator in the nursing program at a College. Mary completed the Palliative Approach to Care program and Fundamentals of Palliative Care course. She is a specialized Registered Nurse who delivers care to patients with life-limiting progressive illnesses using an evidence-based holistic approach to care. She is currently employed in the area in which she believes she can make the most difference, as a Palliative Care Nurse. She has found her true calling and passion working with palliative patients and their families, all of whom continue to inspire her each and every day. Mary lives in Canada with her husband and children.

CPSIA information can be obtained
at www.ICGtesting.com
Printed in the USA
LVHW02s0110160318
569901LV00003B/3/P